COPING WITH PARKINSON DISEASE

The Complete Guide to Managing Your Symptoms for Patients Living with Parkinson Disease, their Loved Ones, and Caregivers

Dr. C. ROLAND

CHAPTER ONE

Introduction

Parkinson's disease is a neurological condition that mostly impairs movement. It was named after Dr. James Parkinson, who originally characterized the illness in 1817, and has since become the focus of much research and awareness. This introduction attempts to lay the groundwork for readers new to Parkinson's disease, providing insights into its nature, symptoms, and the critical role of good care in improving the quality of life for patients and their support networks.

Understanding Parkinson's Disease

Parkinson's disease is a degenerative neurological

condition that predominantly affects dopamine-producing neurons in the brain. Dopamine is a neurotransmitter that controls movement and coordination. When these neurons are injured or die, the brain fails to create enough dopamine, resulting in the classic symptoms of Parkinson's disease.

Tremors, stiffness, sluggish mobility, and postural instability are some of the most common symptoms. While these motor symptoms are characteristic, Parkinson's disease can also cause cognitive abnormalities, emotional issues, and autonomic dysfunction. Understanding the varied nature of Parkinson's disease is critical for both patients and caregivers, allowing for a more complete approach to management.

Overview of Symptoms and Progression

Parkinson's Disease symptoms can vary greatly between individuals, and their progression is frequently unique to each patient. Early stages may include minor tremors or changes in handwriting, however advanced stages might result in major mobility issues and cognitive impairment. It is critical to understand that the course of Parkinson's disease is unpredictable, and symptoms may change over time.

The disease progresses slowly and is separated into stages, allowing healthcare practitioners to analyze and treat patients' changing needs.

Understanding the progression of Parkinson's disease allows people and their caregivers to anticipate and plan for anticipated obstacles, supporting a proactive and informed approach to care.

Importance of Proper Management: Parkinson's disease must be managed properly in order to reduce symptoms, maintain independence, and improve general well-being. While there is no cure for Parkinson's disease, there are a variety of treatment options and methods available to help manage the symptoms.

Early diagnosis and intervention are critical in improving management outcomes. Medications, physical and occupational therapy, and lifestyle changes can all help improve a patient's quality of life. Furthermore, a holistic approach that takes into account both motor and non-motor symptoms, as well as the emotional and psychological aspects of the condition, is critical for delivering thorough care.

This book will go deeper into these topics, providing practical advice, insights, and support for patients, loved ones, and caregivers as they navigate the intricacies of Parkinson's disease.

Recognizing Early Symptoms

Parkinson's disease is a progressive neurological ailment that frequently manifests with modest symptoms, and early detection of these symptoms is critical for obtaining prompt medical assistance. While symptoms differ from person to person, being aware of common early warning signals can assist individuals and their loved ones in taking proactive efforts toward diagnosis and treatment.

1. Tremors:

Parkinson's disease is characterized by tremors, sometimes known as shaking. They typically begin on one side of the body, usually in the hands, fingers, or even the chin. These tremors may appear at rest and subside with deliberate movement.

2. Bradykinesia (slow movement):

• Parkinson's disease patients may experience slowing of their movements over time. This can have an impact on daily activities such as walking, dressing, and doing tasks requiring fine motor skills.

3. Muscle stiffness, or rigidity:

• Early warning signs include muscle stiffness, especially in the arms or legs. This rigidity can make movement unpleasant and contribute to a limited range of motion.

4. Postural instability:

• Problems with balance and coordination may emerge. Individuals may be more prone to stumbling or having difficulties keeping an upright position, which increases the risk of falling.

5. Changes in handwriting

• Parkinson's illness can impact fine motor abilities, resulting in handwriting alterations. "Micrographia," or small, cramped handwriting, is a frequent observation.

6. Reduced Facial Expression:

• A diminution in facial expressions, known as "masked face," may develop. This makes the person's face appear less active, and they may struggle to communicate emotions through facial movements.

7. Changed Walking Patterns:

• Walking changes, such as shuffling or reduced arm swing, may be visible. Individuals may struggle to commence or complete tasks smoothly.

8. Soft or monotone speech:

Parkinson's disease may damage speech muscles, resulting in a quieter or monotone voice. This can reduce communication clarity and expressiveness.

9. Microscopic Hand Movements:

• Resting tremor refers to tiny, regular movements in the hands or fingers that are more evident at rest.

Recognizing these early warning signals demands paying attention to changes in one's own or a loved one's body. While these symptoms can be ascribed to a variety of sources, persistent or worsening problems should prompt a visit to a healthcare practitioner for a thorough evaluation. Seeking medical counsel early in the process can help with rapid diagnosis and the implementation of suitable management methods to improve quality of life and slow the progression of the condition.

Seeking a Diagnosis: Medical Tests and Evaluation.

When early indications and symptoms of Parkinson's disease are identified, a thorough medical evaluation is required to determine a diagnosis. A neurologist, a doctor who specializes in nervous system problems, is usually the primary healthcare expert involved in the diagnosis.

1. Medical History Review:

- A thorough evaluation of a person's medical history is the first step towards a diagnosis. The neurologist will inquire about the start, progression, and type of the symptoms, as well as any pertinent family medical history.

2. Physical Exam:

- A neurological examination evaluates motor abilities, strength, reflexes, and coordination. The neurologist analyzes movements, looks for tremors, and assesses other physical characteristics that may indicate Parkinson's disease.

3. Diagnostic Tests:

- Imaging studies (MRI or CT Scan) can rule out other illnesses that may be similar to Parkinson's disease. They give detailed images of the brain, allowing healthcare practitioners to detect any anatomical abnormalities.

• DaTscan: A specialized imaging technique for assessing dopamine levels in the brain. It can help confirm the loss of dopamine-producing cells, which is a hallmark of Parkinson's disease.

• Blood tests may be performed to rule out other medical disorders causing symptoms similar to Parkinson's disease, as there is no specific test for this condition.

4. Response to Medication:

• Positive responses to Parkinson's drugs may further support a diagnosis. Neurologists may prescribe a trial of Parkinson's drugs to see if symptoms improve.

5. Collaboration With Specialists:

- Additional specialists, such as movement disorder specialists, neurosurgeons, or physical therapists, may be consulted based on the symptoms presented to aid in diagnosis.

6. Second Opinions:

Getting a second opinion might be beneficial, particularly for complex conditions like Parkinson's disease. Another neurologist's opinion may provide new information and result in a more accurate diagnosis.

Understanding the Emotional Impact of Diagnosis.

Receiving a Parkinson's disease diagnosis is a life-changing event that can elicit a wide range of emotions in both the diagnosed individual and their loved ones. Understanding and managing the emotional impact of the diagnosis is critical for developing resilience, successful coping, and general well-being.

1. Shock and denial:

• Initial Reaction: Receiving a Parkinson's diagnosis might cause shock and disbelief. It might take time for people to accept the reality of their situation, leading to a period of denial as they deal with the consequences of living with a chronic ailment.

• Healthcare professionals and support networks should approach individuals with empathy, understanding that shock and denial are common reactions. Encourage open conversation and provide clear information about the condition to assist people progressively accept their diagnosis.

2. F ear and Anxiety:

• Uncertainty regarding Parkinson's disease development might lead to fear and anxiety. Individuals may be concerned about how their symptoms may progress, how it will affect their daily lives, and the potential problems they will encounter.

• Coping Strategy: Education can help reduce fear and anxiety. Healthcare practitioners should take the time to explain Parkinson's disease, its typical development, and treatment options. Providing a blueprint for the path ahead can help people face the future with more confidence.

3. Grief and loss:

• Adjusting Expectations: A Parkinson's diagnosis typically necessitates adjusting one's expectations and plans for the future. The knowledge that life may not go as planned might cause feelings of grief and loss.

• Coping Strategy: Recognizing grief is crucial. Healthcare experts, counselors, and support groups can help people express their emotions and work through the transition to a new normal. Encouraging people to focus on what they can control and seek out new sources of fulfillment might be good.

4. Impact on Relationships:

• Parkinson's disease can impair speech and physical abilities, potentially affecting relationships with family and friends. Maintaining open channels of communication is critical for addressing potential issues and avoiding feelings of isolation.

• Education on Parkinson's disease and its impact on relationships is essential for coping strategy. Encouraging relatives and friends to attend support groups or counseling sessions might help them understand and develop their ties. Effective communication strategies, such as adopting different forms of expression, can also be investigated.

5. Connecting with support:

• Connecting with those who understand Parkinson's can alleviate the emotional stress of the diagnosis. In-person and online support groups can provide a significant sense of belonging and understanding.

• Early access to support networks can help individuals cope with their diagnoses. Healthcare providers can advise patients about local support groups, internet forums, and other services that allow them to connect with others who are facing similar issues.

6. Mental Health Support:

• Addressing Depression and Anxiety: A Parkinson's diagnosis can lead to emotional issues, including depression and anxiety. Recognizing and treating these difficulties is critical to overall well-being.

- Integrating mental health support into the care plan is vital. Referrals to therapists or counselors with experience in chronic illness can help people manage the emotional complexity of Parkinson's disease.

CHAPTER TWO

Treatment Options for Parkinson's Disease

1. Medications For Symptom Control

Parkinson's disease is essentially defined by a lack of dopamine, a neurotransmitter that is essential for controlling movement. Medications are designed to ease symptoms by either replacing or replicating dopamine's effects. Commonly prescribed drugs include:

Levodopa:

• Converts into dopamine in the brain to refill depleted amounts.

• Effective in relieving motor symptoms such as tremors and stiffness.

Dopamine agonists:

• The mechanism mimics the activity of dopamine in the brain.

• Effective in controlling motor symptoms and can be administered alongside or instead of levodopa.

MAO-B inhibitors:

• The mechanism involves blocking the enzyme that breaks down dopamine to increase its levels.

• Effect: Can be used alone or with other drugs.

COMT inhibitors:

• Prolongs the benefits of levodopa by preventing its breakdown.

- Improves the duration of symptom alleviation when used with levodopa.

Anticholinergics:

- The mechanism involves blocking acetylcholine to balance neurotransmitters in the brain.

- Effect: Treats tremors and other motor disorders.

Effective drug management frequently entails determining the optimal combination and dosage based on the individual's needs. Regular follow-ups with healthcare specialists are essential for monitoring and adjusting the treatment strategy as the condition advances.

2. Surgical intervention with deep brain stimulation (DBS)

In circumstances where drugs alone do not give enough symptom relief, surgical treatments, including Deep Brain Stimulation (DBS), may be considered.

DBS procedure:

• The procedure involves implanting electrodes in specific parts of the brain.

• The electrodes emit electrical impulses that modulate aberrant neural activity.

• Results: Significant reduction in motor symptoms, particularly tremors and dyskinesias.

DBS is often advised for people who have Parkinson's disease for a long time and have difficulty controlling their symptoms with medicines. While DBS can not cure Parkinson's disease, it can enhance quality of life by allowing for more consistent and dependable symptom management.

3. Complementary therapies include physical and occupational therapy.

Complementary therapies, notably physical and occupational therapy, can help manage Parkinson's disease by addressing both motor and non-motor symptoms.

Physical therapy:

• Priority: Enhancing mobility, balance, and total physical function.

• Exercises focus on specific muscle areas, coordination, and flexibility.

- Benefits: Reduces gait irregularities, improves posture, and decreases the chance of falling.

Occupational therapy:

- Goal: Improve independence in daily tasks.

- Adaptations to home surroundings, assistive devices, and approaches to improve daily chores.

- Benefits: Enhances quality of life by promoting independence and reducing the impact of motor and non-motor symptoms on everyday activities.

Including these medicines early in the treatment plan can considerably improve the functional abilities and overall well-being of Parkinson's patients.

A multidisciplinary healthcare team, including of neurologists, physical therapists, and occupational therapists, must work together to develop an effective and thorough treatment plan. Regular communication and revisions to the treatment plan ensure that the strategy remains consistent with the individual's changing demands throughout the course of Parkinson's disease.

Lifestyle Strategies for Patients with Parkinson's Disease

Living with Parkinson's disease entails not just treating symptoms with drugs and therapies, but also implementing lifestyle changes that promote general well-being. These tactics include nutrition, exercise, cognitive and mental health maintenance, and practical advice for everyday life.

1. Nutrition and Exercise: A Holistic Approach

> **Maintain a balanced diet.**

• Prioritize a balanced diet including fruits, vegetables, lean meats, and whole grains.

• Benefits: Promotes general health, aids in weight management, and delivers necessary minerals. Some people may benefit from a dietitian's advice to meet specific nutritional requirements.

> **Hydration:**

• Importance: Staying hydrated is vital for everyone, especially those with Parkinson's disease who may struggle to swallow.

• Practical Tip: Drinking water throughout the day helps maintain hydrated without straining the digestive system.

> **Exercise routine:**

• Types: Combine aerobic exercises (e.g. walking, cycling) with strength training.

• Improves flexibility, balance, and muscle strength, reducing motor symptoms and the risk of falls.

• Make fitness a habit by engaging in enjoyable activities.

2. Cognitive and mental health maintenance

❖ **Mental stimulation:**

• Engage in mentally stimulating hobbies like puzzles, reading, and acquiring new skills.

• Benefits: Improves cognitive health and may aid in managing non-motor symptoms including cognitive decline and dementia.

❖ **Social engagement:**

• Importance: Maintaining social relationships is crucial for emotional health.

• Engage in social activities, support groups, and maintain regular contact with friends and family.

• Tip: Plan activities based on your hobbies, such as a reading club, art class, or support group.

❖ **Stress management:**

- Use stress-reduction strategies including deep breathing, meditation, and yoga.

- Benefits include managing non-motor symptoms such as anxiety and improving general well-being.

3. Practical Tips for Daily Life

> **Adaptive devices:**

- Use tools and technologies to help with daily chores, such as adaptable utensils, grab bars, and mobility aids.

- Benefits: Improves independence by making daily duties more achievable.

> **Structured routine:**

- Establishing a regular routine promotes predictability and stability.

• Practical Tip: Plan activities and breaks carefully, prioritizing key tasks during optimal energy and symptom control.

> **Proper Sleep Hygiene:**

• Practices: Stick to a steady sleep schedule, create a relaxing sleep environment, and avoid stimulants before bedtime.

• Quality sleep improves physical and mental health, reducing symptoms and improving overall function.

Parkinson's Disease Patient Support Systems

1. Creating a Strong Healthcare Team

Neurologist:

• Parkinson's sufferers typically seek primary treatment from a neurologist who specializes in movement disorders. They diagnose, prescribe drugs, and oversee the overall therapy approach.

• Regular follow-ups with the neurologist allow for continuing assessment and modifications to the treatment plan based on the individual's changing needs.

Specialized therapists:

• Physical and occupational therapists help maintain mobility, balance, and independence with targeted exercises and adaptive strategies.

• Speech therapists address communication and swallowing issues.

Mental Health Professions:

• Psychiatrists and psychologists assist emotional well-being, including treating mood disorders, anxiety, and depression.

• Counselors provide coping strategies, stress management techniques, and a safe space for people and families to address emotional difficulties.

A multidisciplinary healthcare team provides comprehensive care by addressing both the physical and emotional components of Parkinson's disease.

2. Connecting to Support Groups

➤ Local Support Groups:

• Joining local Parkinson's support groups might help you connect with others facing similar issues.

• Sharing experiences, insights, and resources helps build a sense of community and understanding.

> Online Support Communities:

• Online forums and social media groups provide global accessibility to the Parkinson's community.

• Online communities offer 24/7 assistance for anyone seeking guidance, encouragement, or information.

> Patient Advocacy Organizations:

• The Parkinson's Foundation and Michael J. Fox Foundation provide educational tools for patients and caregivers, including webinars.

- Advocacy Opportunities: Participating in advocacy initiatives can help individuals contribute to the Parkinson's community and promote awareness.

Connecting with support groups creates a network of empathy and encouragement, alleviating feelings of loneliness and providing practical insights.

3. The Function of Family and Friends in the Coping Process

❖ Emotional Support:

• Family and friends can provide emotional support for those with Parkinson's disease by recognizing the obstacles they experience.

• Active listening without judgment enables individuals to

communicate their feelings and worries freely.

❖ **Practical Assistance:**

• Assistance with daily tasks, including meal preparation, transportation, and household chores, can greatly reduce the load on Parkinson's patients.

• Accompanying medical appointments helps relay critical information and provide additional assistance.

❖ **Educational involvement:**

• Educating oneself on Parkinson's disease helps family and friends comprehend the condition and actively participate in management plans.

• Participation in therapies, such as physical and occupational therapy or support groups, fosters shared experiences and understanding.

Creating a supportive environment within the family and friend circle improves the general well-being of Parkinson's patients. Clear communication, empathy, and active participation in the coping process all help to build a better support system.

Coping Mechanisms for Loved Ones of Patients with Parkinson's

1. Understanding and Managing Caregivers' Stress

Recognition of Stressors:

• Identifying problems: Loved ones should identify the various problems connected with caregiving, including the emotional, physical, and logistical components.

• Monitoring personal well-being is essential for maintaining good mental and physical health. Regular self-assessment aids in detecting indicators of stress early on.

Seeking Support:

• Joining caregiver support groups can help exchange experiences and coping skills with others facing similar issues.

• Professional counseling provides a discreet environment to examine the emotional effects of caregiving and build effective coping mechanisms.

Taking breaks:

• Caregivers can avoid burnout by scheduling respite care or taking breaks as required.

• Setting aside personal time for hobbies or relaxation can help maintain a balanced and fulfilling life outside caregiving responsibilities.

2. Balancing Caregiver Responsibilities

Establishing a routine:

• Creating a schedule helps organize caregiving duties and ensures critical obligations are met consistently.

• Prioritizing Tasks: Identifying and prioritizing tasks helps manage time effectively and prevents feeling overwhelmed.

Delegating tasks:

- Involving family and friends in caring helps distribute responsibilities and provide additional assistance.

- Hiring professional caregivers or utilizing home health services can help manage caregiving responsibilities.

Setting realistic expectations:

- Recognizing personal limitations and setting reasonable expectations can reduce emotions of inadequacy and failure.

- Flexibility: Adapting plans and techniques as needed promotes realistic and sustainable caregiving.

3. Effective Communication with a Loved One with Parkinson's Disease

a) Active Listening:

• Actively listening to individuals with Parkinson's promotes open communication and comprehension of their needs and concerns.

• Empathy: Acknowledging others' emotions and experiences fosters a supportive environment.

b) Clear Communication:

• Clear and straightforward language improves comprehension, particularly for individuals with cognitive impairments.

• Encouraging Expression: Creating a comfortable environment for individuals to express their feelings and needs leads to good communication.

Including Them in Decision Making:

• Involving individuals in care discussions and decision-making fosters empowerment and a sense of control.

• Respecting Independence: Maintaining dignity by balancing support and independence.

Implementing these coping methods not only improves the well-being of loved ones caring for people with Parkinson's disease, but it also leads to a more supportive and understanding connection between caregivers and those they care for. Balancing caregiving obligations, finding support, and promoting effective communication are all necessary components of a long-term and positive caregiving experience.

CHAPTER THREE

Emotional Wellbeing in Parkinson's Disease

1. Addressing Depression and Anxiety

i.   Recognition of Symptoms:

• Awareness: Parkinson's patients and loved ones should recognize indicators of depression and anxiety, including chronic melancholy, changes in sleep patterns, and emotions of worry.

• Healthcare practitioners should conduct regular examinations for mood disorders during medical checkups.

ii.   Professional Interventions:

• Seeking support from psychiatrists, psychologists, or counselors who specialize in chronic conditions can give specialized interventions.

• Medications may be administered to address depression or anxiety symptoms.

iii. Participation in Support groups:

• Support groups provide opportunities to exchange experiences, coping skills, and emotional support with others facing similar issues.

• Validating emotions in a group context promotes a sense of belonging and reduces isolation.

2. Developing resilience and a positive mindset

1) Mindfulness and meditation:

• Deep breathing and meditation are mindfulness techniques that can relieve stress by focusing on the present moment.

• Incorporating positive affirmations into daily practices can foster a more optimistic outlook.

2) Gratitude Practices:

• Keeping a gratitude journal can help focus on positive parts of life.

• Reflecting on pleasant events on a daily basis can improve one's outlook.

3) Engaging in Hobbies and Activities:

• Pursuing enjoyable hobbies and activities can give a beneficial distraction from emotional issues.

• Social connection: Spending time with loved ones develops friendships and improves emotional well-being.

3. Exploring Therapeutic Approaches to Emotional Support

a) Counseling and psychotherapy:

• Individual Therapy: One-on-one counseling offers a personalized environment to explore emotions, coping skills, and stress management.

• Cognitive-Behavioral Therapy (CBT) can effectively treat negative thought patterns and promote positive cognitive processes.

b) Art and Music Therapy:

• Art and music therapy provide creative channels for emotional expression and can be beneficial for people with Parkinson's.

• Stress Reduction: Research indicates that these therapies can reduce stress and promote emotional well-being.

c) Pet therapy:

• Interacting with pets can relieve stress and increase happiness. The company of a pet can be especially reassuring.

Incorporating a combination of these emotional well-being measures into one's daily routine helps to promote a comprehensive approach to Parkinson's disease management. Addressing emotional issues, building resilience, and exploring therapeutic options all contribute to a more pleasant and fulfilling quality of life for Parkinson's patients and their families.

Planning for the Future: Parkinson's Disease

1. Legal and Financial Considerations

❖ Advanced directives:

• A living will and healthcare proxy define an individual's medical treatment preferences in case they are unable to communicate their wishes.

• Power of Attorney: A trusted individual can make financial decisions for someone with Parkinson's if they are unable to manage their own affairs.

❖ Estate Planning:

• Creating a will and trusts ensures asset distribution and clarifies individual intentions.

• Regularly monitoring and revising beneficiary designations on financial accounts and insurance policies is important.

❖ Insurance Coverage:

• Managing medical bills requires complete health insurance coverage and an awareness of policy details.

• Consider long-term care insurance to cover payments for extended care needs.

2. Long-term Care Planning

❖ Home Modifications:

• Modifying the home with handrails, ramps, and bathrooms improves mobility and safety.

• Utilizing assistive devices, such mobility assistance or home automation, can improve freedom and comfort.

❖ Caregiver Support:

• Planning for professional caregiving help, such as in-home care or assisted living facilities, may be important as the condition develops.

• Respite Care: Providing respite care choices helps primary caregivers take breaks and minimize burnout.

❖ Daytime Programs and Activities:

• Engaging in Parkinson's-specific day programs offers social, cognitive, and community benefits.

3. Navigating the Advanced Stages of Parkinson's Disease

➢ Hospice and Palliative Care:

• Moving to hospice or palliative care in advanced stages prioritizes quality of life, symptom management, and emotional support.

• End-of-Life Discussions: Communicating with healthcare providers and loved ones about end-of-life preferences helps match with individual wishes.

➢ Emotional support for families:

- Grief counseling and support groups can help families cope with the emotional challenges of severe Parkinson's disease.

- Regular family gatherings promote open communication and ensure consensus on caring decisions and end-of-life desires.

  ➢ Legacy Planning:

- Encouraging individuals with Parkinson's to document their experiences, wishes, and personal stories can create a lasting legacy.

- Family Discussions: Engaging family members in discussions about the individual's life and legacy promotes connection and understanding.

Future planning must be approached with flexibility, with plans revisited and adjusted on a regular basis to reflect changing demands and circumstances. Collaboration with legal and financial specialists, healthcare providers, and support networks ensures that Parkinson's disease patients receive a complete and tailored approach to future planning.

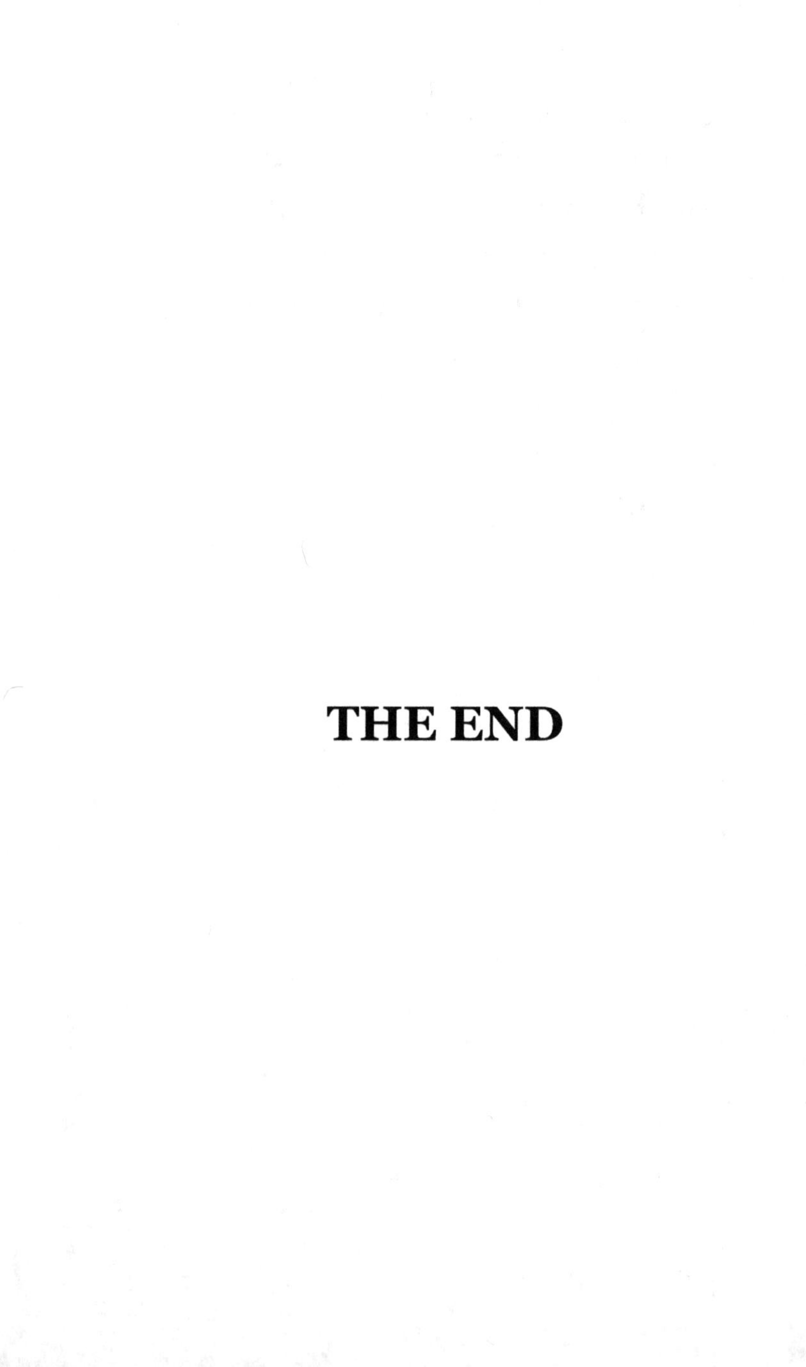

THE END